COCONUT OIL AND
APPLE CIDER VINEGAR

RAPID WEIGHT LOSS AND ULTIMATE HEATH WITH MOTHER NATURE'S NECTARS

By Darrin Wiggins

Download Your Thank You Gifts

Are You Someone Who Wants To Be Healthy, Wealthy And Happy?

Subscribe to get alerts when our eBooks have flash sales for 99-cents and even free. Collect all of your favorite eBooks from the following bestselling authors for just a "buck" each or less

- Health, Fitness & Weight Loss with Darrin Wiggins

- Personal Development & Self-Help with Seth Cohen

- Delicious Recipes For Any Dietary Lifestyle with Charity Wilson

- Receive the FREE eBooks: Lifestyle Design Mastery plus the eBook 100 Weight Loss Tips That Work With Any Diet

Just follow the link below to get access

www.inspiringhealthwealthandhappiness.com

Table of Contents

The Miracle of Coconut Oil

The Western world is only recently catching on, but coconut oil has been used by those in the Philippines, India, Pakistan, Indonesia, Sri Lanka and other Southeast Asian countries for decades as an astonishingly versatile food, medicine, and beauty aid. There is virtually nothing that coconut oil can't help you with, and we'll be looking at some of the most popular uses – including, of course, how coconut oil can help you lose weight.

Let's start at the beginning. Coconuts grow on the wonderfully tropical-looking coco palm tree in clusters. Baby coconuts, or "jelly nuts", are soft and can be eaten whole, and the outside fibers of mature coconuts can be woven into rugs, nets, and ropes. Inside, the coconut water is a healthy and delicious drink, and the coconut "meat" can be dried and scraped out to make "copra" which is often used as animal feed.

The "good stuff", however, is the coconut flesh that is wet milled and processed to extract the precious oil. It takes a thousand coconuts – that's over 3000 pounds – to make 370 pounds of copra which is then turned into 18 gallons of smooth, white, delicious coconut oil.

So, what's so special about coconut oil?

For those convinced of its benefits, coconut oil is like mother's milk – almost literally. Coconut oil contains lauric acid, which the body converts to Monolaurin, a molecule only found in one other place – human breast milk. Other than being more than 50% Lauric acid, coconut oil also contains Caprylic acid, Decanoic acid, and Palmitic acid.

These are all saturated, medium chain fatty acids which are what makes coconut oil so unique. These medium-chain triglycerides or MCTs, differ from the longer chain acids in other oils in that they don't require much digestion for the body to absorb. What's more, MCTs have been shown in several studies to aid in weight loss.

Coconut oil is renowned as a potent natural antiviral, antifungal, antibiotic, and antimicrobial. Coconut oil dissolves the outer protective coating on viruses and bacteria and kills them, while also being able to rebalance intestinal flora, suffocate head lice, and destroy microbes on the surface of the skin – among many other things!

Are all coconut oils the same?

Unfortunately not. Depending on where in the extraction process your oil originates, and what has been added or removed, coconut oils can vary greatly in quality. A poor quality oil will be largely useless or – worse – toxic. Here's how to make sense of coconut oil labels so you can buy the right kind.

Virgin Coconut Oil

The World Health Organization has industry standards for the proper processing of fresh, mature coconuts into virgin coconut oil. At a bare minimum, the oil you buy should be virgin, although don't fall for marketing tricks like the label "extra virgin", which is meaningless. There is no difference between virgin and extra virgin coconut oil according to Health Impact News.

You need your oil to be unrefined and unhydrogenated (some brands are hydrogenated to make sure they're solid at warmer temperatures). Organic oil is great if you can find it although not absolutely necessary in order to derive the full health benefits. Lastly, "raw" coconut oil is also something of a gimmick as almost all coconut oil is processed with some heat at one point or another; the correct heat does not affect the oil's quality. Good coconut oil should have a pleasant, rich, nutty taste of actual coconuts and no hint of chemical residue.

Refined, Bleached and Deodorized (RBD)

If you're unsure about a coconut oil, give it a sniff. If it's "RBD" coconut oil, it will have been processed more extensively than virgin oil to remove the odor. Virgin coconut oil will still smell like coconuts. While this type of oil is not really suitable for eating straight from the jar or in large quantities, it's still valuable for cosmetic use or cooking and baking where you don't necessarily want the taste of coconut overpowering everything. It's also a lot cheaper, so it makes a good choice when you need some coconut oil but don't want to splash out on the more expensive kind.

Hydrogenated Oils

Avoid these at all costs. The hydrogenation process converts some of those healthful fatty acids into harmful trans fatty acids. By heating the oil and adding a hydrogen atom (hence the name), companies can benefit from longer shelf life and an oil that doesn't melt. The process is done for commercial reasons and not for anyone's health. Again: avoid. Hydrogenated oil will be quite firm and have a texture similar to hard margarine.

Other things to look out for: Coconut oil should be very obviously white so skip any if the color isn't right. The price is also a good indication of quality. Expect to pay around $15 for a 16-oz jar and be suspicious if it's very much less than that. If you can, go to a health food store and chat with the owner about where they get their oil and what quality it is.

Some people claim that glass jars retain flavor and nutrition better than plastic ones, although this may be a personal preference. Lastly, don't be swayed by pretty pictures or the fact that a brand of coconut oil is available at a health food store – study the label carefully before you buy!

Highly rated coconut oils

Choosing a good oil can be a bit bewildering – but here are 3 popular and good quality oils currently available for sale on Amazon.com:

1. Nutiva Organic Extra Virgin Coconut Oil

2. Trader Joe's Organic Virgin Coconut Oil

3. Nature's Way Organic Coconut Oil

If cost is an issue, you might choose to go for a cheaper, refined oil for cosmetic use and get the best quality oil for everything else. If you can afford it, however, organic, unrefined, virgin coconut oil is always best.

How do I store coconut oil?

Coconut oil oxidizes at an incredibly slow rate, meaning it won't go rancid if you just leave it be. It doesn't need to be refrigerated and can be kept in a cool, dry place for up to two years before going bad. In cold weather, however, coconut oil will solidify.

In warmer weather, coconut oil will soften and even liquefy. At room temperature it's usually a solid, crumbly white fat similar in appearance to lard. If you need to spread it, you could simply warm the oil between your palms (if you intend to apply it to the skin) or gently melt it in a double boiler. Avoid melting in the microwave.

Darrin Wiggins

Health and Beauty Benefits of Coconut Oil

We've had a look at what coconut oil is and where to find the best kinds. Now, when it comes to the benefits of coconut oil, it's difficult to know where to start. Coconut oil is so mild on the skin, so easy to digest, and so full of vitamins, minerals, and healing fats that the entire body can probably benefit from it in some way. Before we get to the specific reasons coconut oil can help you melt away fat, let's look at the many other ways coconut oil can improve your life.

Coconut Oil: Beauty in a Bottle

This luxurious oil is packed with lipids and phospholipids that bathe the skin in healing, soothing moisture. Coconut oil also contains vitamins E and K, and its antiviral, antifungal, and antimicrobial powers make it an excellent ointment for athlete's foot, rashes of all kinds, cuts, burns, and scrapes.

There's no real secret to using coconut oil externally – simply apply. The oil is silky and easily absorbed, and will leave your skin supple and soft and smelling like a tropical island. In fact, many people rely solely on coconut oil as their skin care regime. After washing the face with nothing but water and gentle exfoliation, the skin is massaged with a small bead of the oil. Coconut oil makes a great moisturizer, but should be applied sparingly – it's so rich that it can clog pores if applied excessively.

Try this for a coconut oil-themed spa you can do at home: Hop in the shower and scrub down your entire body with an equal mix of coconut oil, granulated sugar, and a teaspoon of powdered cinnamon. Use firm but gentle strokes to slough off dead skin cells – the cinnamon and coconut oil will encourage blood flow and leave you feeling rosy and glowing. Afterwards, apply a generous amount of coconut oil over your body to seal in moisture. This treatment can fade scars and stretch marks, soothe dry skin and eczema, calm irritation, and leave your skin elastic and gleaming with health.

But you needn't stop there. Coconut oil does wonders for the hair as well. The oil is capable of coating each strand and so prevents damage caused by friction. The fatty acids in the oil meld together the hair proteins and strengthen the molecular structure, making it ideal for pampering color-treated or over-processed hair.

Coconut oil leaves a very thin residue over the entire head, scalp, and every strand of hair. This offers protection from the sun and pollution, while sealing in moisture and leaving your hair feeling heavy and easy to manage. What's more, the antifungal effects of coconut oil banish microorganisms from the surface of the scalp and can heal and soothe hair follicles. This is important because infections of the scalp and follicles are a common cause of dandruff, dryness, and hair loss. By cleansing the skin of parasites and simultaneously soothing the skin, coconut oil leaves you with a healthy scalp. And a healthy scalp means healthy hair!

Here's a hair treatment for all your hair woes: Apply enough liquid coconut oil to coat the entire head and each hair thoroughly. Wrap or braid the hair and cover with a shower cap and a towel on top of that to encourage warmth. Leave on for a minimum of an hour, overnight if possible. You can then comb out and wash your hair. It will be soft and shiny and will feel nourished. Add to this a few drops of essential oils and you'll not only feel great, you'll smell heavenly, too.

Expectant mothers will find coconut oil to be an excellent twice-daily massage oil that will leave them with a real pregnancy glow and help prevent the development of stretch marks. You can also make your own coconut shampoo by combining castile soap flakes, coconut milk, a bit of coconut oil, and a few drops of rosemary oil. Wash and rinse, then follow with a diluted apple cider vinegar rinse. You can even use coconut oil as a light styling cream by applying it to fly-aways or split ends. During the winter – when static electricity can wreak havoc with your hair – a tiny coating of coconut oil can prevent damage and keep things slick.

If you can think of a place on your body to put coconut oil, go ahead and put some there. Rub a little into the lips to make a lip balm – or even your own lip gloss by adding food coloring, beet juice, or red mica powder. Use it for razor burns and diaper rashes, mosquito bites or rosacea, varicose veins, age spots, as a makeup remover or on sunburn. Rub it into cracked heels and cover with a sock for the night – you'll be amazed the next morning at how smooth your skin feels there. Of course, it can also smooth out rough elbows and hands. And – just in case you were wondering – coconut oil can be used as a personal lubricant, too!

Not just for a pretty face.

Coconut oil is a champion moisturizer, but it really shines as a health food in its own right. By working on every system in your body, coconut oil is a surprisingly effective holistic health tonic.

Candida Albicans is a nasty, parasitic yeast-like fungus that lives in the intestinal tract in small quantities. However, imbalances in the hormone levels or immune system deficiencies can mean that sometimes the body allows the Candida population to get out of hand. Candida damages the cells of the intestinal walls, allowing harmful digestive particles to enter into your bloodstream and cause a whole host of problems.

Candida is responsible for thrush of all kinds and, when an overgrowth occurs, can cause a number of unpleasant symptoms. Because the immune system is exhausted trying to fight this constant low-grade infection, it becomes oversensitive and, accordingly, you may suffer from the "false positive" of seasonal allergies. Your body produces histamines in response to perceived threat and you may experience hay fever or food sensitivities.

Candida overgrowth can affect your digestion and absorption, leaving you bloated, depressed, anxious, fatigued, and susceptible to frequent infections. You may suffer vaginal thrush and cold sores, get chilly easily, and generally feel fat and under the weather.

Here's where coconut oil can come to the rescue. By breaking down the walls of those nasty little Candida cells, coconut oil gives your body the chance to repopulate the gut with beneficial bacteria. It's full of soothing lipids that speed healing of the gastrointestinal lining and create a seal against further infection. Coconut oil also has the ability to correct both diarrhea and constipation because of its calming effect on the gastrointestinal tract.

Candida isn't the only organism that hates living with coconut oil. Many viruses and parasites are similarly damaged by the fatty acids in the oil, particularly helicobacter pylori, which is responsible for more than its fair share of Irritable Bowel Syndrome symptoms and weight gain.

Coconut oil and arthritis

Coconut oil's superhero powers as a viral and fungal fighter also applies to places you might not have considered, for example, the body's joints. Many doctors are beginning to discover that inflammation of the joints and certain types of arthritis are caused by infection. The trouble is antibiotics do not seem particularly useful at eradicating joint infection.

Why? Well, the joints are special in that they aren't bathed in their own bloodstream like other body parts. The joints are sealed in their own individual membranes, and neither blood nor antibiotics in the blood, can easily penetrate these membranes. But coconut oil can. By both consuming coconut oil internally, and applying it externally, the medium-chain fatty acids in coconut oil dissolve and get to work killing infections in painful joints.

Make coconut oil part of your arthritis regime by massaging the area daily and taking up to 3 tablespoons of best-quality oil daily. The healing lipids and vitamins heat up and lubricate the joint from the outside and, from the inside, harmful infections are killed off.

Even if you don't suffer from arthritis, you can take advantage of coconut oil's anti-inflammatory powers. Massage tired or sore muscles with coconut oil, even adding a few drops of other essential oils. Camphor and lavender are excellent for this purpose. Sprains, aches, and overtrained muscles can all be loosened, warmed, and relieved. Coconut oil increases blood flow and delivers antioxidants and anti-inflammatories directly into the affected area.

Coconut oil: Good for just about everything

Cuts will often heal faster with an application of coconut oil as the film it creates forms a natural barrier against dust and further infection, all the while speeding connective tissue repair. Coconut oil is also great for hemorrhoids because it's a good source of fiber in the diet and because it soothes the inflamed area. By balancing the intestinal flora and encouraging peristalsis, coconut oil regulates diarrhea and constipation, meaning less strain and so fewer hemorrhoids.

Ingest coconut oil to relieve heartburn, too. The oil neutralizes and calms acid in the esophagus, soothing digestion and reducing the chance that the stomach will over-produce acid. At the same time, the oil coats and calms the inner linings and repairs damage at the cellular level.

Finally, coconut oil is great for all bone conditions as it enhances calcium and magnesium absorption, benefitting the teeth and the bones of those healing a fracture as well as for women over the age of 50 who may suffer from calcium deficiency. Some nutritionists even claim that regular consumption of coconut oil is able to remineralize the teeth and repair cavities by allowing the tissue to regenerate.

Using coconut oil for a gleaming set of pearly whites

It may seem like a strange thought, but coconut oil can be an excellent tool in your dental health regime. Coconut oil really shines as an all-over healer and nourisher, and this is evident when you consider its power to stop infection at the source – the mouth.

The gums, teeth, and tongue harbor entire colonies of bacteria and microorganisms.

Infections in the mouth can often translate into infection of the rest of the intestinal tract and, eventually, into every system of the body. Brushing and flossing can help to some extent but, for many people, this is simply not enough.

Here is where coconut oil "pulling" comes in. Oil pulling may seem a little strange and off-putting at first, but once you experience the positive results you may grow to love it as a regular healing treatment.

Here's how you do it. First thing in the morning, take up to a tablespoon of good quality coconut oil in your mouth. If it's solid, take a few moments to break it up a little and melt it until it pours freely. Then set your timer for 15 to 20 minutes. What you'll be doing is swishing and swirling the liquid oil all around the inside of your mouth. Have fun with it and send the oil into every nook and cranny, pulsing it through the spaces in your teeth.

Be careful however not to swallow any of the oil. By swishing and swirling, you create millions of tiny bubbles and aerate the oil, allowing it to penetrate everywhere and wash away those harmful particles and microorganisms. The oil dissolves plaque and absorbs the particles responsible for bad breath. Toxins are trapped in the oil – so when you finally spit it out they don't have the chance to enter into your system and cause havoc.

Do oil pulling every day or a few times a week, especially as part of a more intensive coconut oil regimen, and you may notice more energy, fresher breath, and whiter teeth. No matter what ailment you are treating, coconut oil pulling can ensure that you aren't adding to the problem daily by swallowing harmful particles. When you're done pulling, follow by brushing your teeth and doing a mild salt water rinse.

Coconut oil is an amazing immune system booster

We're not quite done yet with the wonders of coconut oil. Because coconut oil eliminates infection in so many different ways, it has the total effect of boosting and strengthening an immune system that is often overtired and overtaxed.

With regular coconut oil pulling, the main entry point for infection can be seriously disrupted. By killing off harmful bacteria in the gut, coconut oil allows the immune system to better protect itself from invasion from the intestinal walls, a massive source of trouble often referred to as a "leaky gut". And by helping with digestion and elimination, coconut oil makes sure your body is as efficient as possible in washing away toxic debris and absorbing nutrients properly.

The result is a body that is better able to resist infection. Here's a tip: A small bit of coconut oil rubbed around the nostrils is a good natural defense during winter when the people around you may be suffering from colds and flu. If you've already contracted something, rub some coconut oil and eucalyptus oil onto your chest and back to relieve stuffiness, or smooth onto red noses that have been worn away with tissues.

A head lice treatment

Here's a quick tip for killing head lice without resorting to harsh and foul smelling shampoos: Drench the entire head and each strand in a jar of coconut oil (yes, a whole jar!), cover with a shower cap and then a towel, and leave on for as long as you can, up to 24 hours. Rinse out and follow with a strong apple cider vinegar rinse (about ½ cup in a jug of water). The oil will dissolve the lice eggs and make it difficult for them to move around, and the vinegar will soften and prevent further infestation. You'll also get a nice hair and scalp treatment in the process.

Coconut oil cleansing for acne

Here's a mild yet effective way to get a handle on facial acne. Morning and night, take 1 teaspoon or less of coconut oil and massage all over a moistened face. Then, using water as hot as you can handle, soak a facecloth and drape over your face for a few moments, holding it against your skin to let the hot steam penetrate into the pores. Don't rub it in. When the cloth cools a little, wet it again and repeat, as many as 5 or 6 times.

The coconut oil combined with the heat will soften your pores, dissolving excess oil and penetrating into old acne scars and dry patches. On the final go, gently massage the remainder of the oil into your face and pat dry with a towel. Follow with a much-diluted apple cider vinegar toner – simply swipe a cotton ball soaked in apple cider vinegar lightly over the T-zone (that area of the face that is most prone to acne). You can make a mixture of 1 teaspoon in about 6 ounces of water. There's no need to moisturize after this.

Other Ways to Use Coconut Oil

• Add to smoothies for a good dose of healthy fats.

• Use to treat, buff and seal leather. Coconut oil is actually excellent at waterproofing shoes from rain and snow.

• A traditional favorite: Use the oil to pop popcorn or as a melted topping.

• Blend or whisk together black coffee, coconut oil, cream, or a milk of any kind with a little cinnamon and vanilla essence for a delicious winter drink.

• Coconut oil dissolves make-up quickly and easily. Swipe a little over your eyelids to remove mascara.

• Use in place of shaving cream that doubles as a moisturizer. The oil will simultaneously moisturize as you shave.

• Add any essential oil to coconut oil and use for massages or rub into dry and ragged cuticles.

• Coconut oil is great for chapped nipples during breastfeeding – and perfectly safe for your baby.

• Add a dollop to bath water for a soothing soak along with Epsom salts, essential oils, and a few sprigs of lavender or rose petals.

• Season cast iron pans or lubricate small machine parts. You only need a little to condition the pan's surface and it will last for years to come.

• Use to remove sticky residues, for example, removing glue left behind by labels. You can also rub coconut oil into knotted hair or remove stuck pieces of gum.

• Feed coconut oil to your dog or cat – they'll benefit the same way you do! Keep it to a minimum, however, since some dogs may experience diarrhea.

Coconut oil certainly has an exhaustive list of benefits. If you are not yet convinced that you need a big barrel of coconut oil in your life, you'll definitely be convinced by the next chapter. We'll look at exactly what makes coconut oil such a champion weight loss aid, and how to start incorporating it into your life right now to become leaner and stronger.

Darrin Wiggins

How Coconut Oil Speeds Weight Loss

Granted, there are quite a few things you can use humble coconut oil for, but what most people are interested in is coconut oil's ability to help them lose weight and burn fat.

For most people, dieting is synonymous with restricting fat. Every magazine, celebrity nutritionist, and old wife encourages us to trim the visible fat off of meat, choose skim milk, and pretend that things like butter and bacon fat simply don't exist.

The advent of both the Atkins diet as well as Paleo eating styles has loosened people's intense fear of fat, although the suspicion remains: If you eat fat, you get fat. Coconut oil is a whopping 86% saturated fat. Just the sound of that is enough to give people heart failure.

In fact, the medical establishment as a whole has, since the 1950s, piled a lot of scorn on saturated fats like coconut oil. Populations that, for centuries, have derived more than half their total calorie intake from coconut oil and who've experienced fewer instances of heart disease and obesity didn't seem to matter.

Instead, doctors warned that too much saturated fat would raise your cholesterol, give you Alzheimer's or heart disease and, of course, make you incredibly fat. As researchers are getting a more sophisticated understanding of different types of saturated fat, however, this misconception is slowly lifting.

Coconut oil is full of medium-chain fatty acids

Most oils contain long-chain fatty acids, which the body has to work hard to break down. By requiring extra enzymes and the processing of by-products to this breaking-down process, these kinds of oils place extra strain on your pancreas, liver, and digestive system. It is these oils that are deposited in the arteries and stored as fat in the body.

Medium chain fatty acids are different, however. The small molecules in coconut oil are easily digested and absorbed. Little to no digestion is required. These fats are preferentially sent to the liver to be used as energy, instead of being stored as adipose tissue. Not only do medium chain fatty acids not make you fat, their special properties actually have the effect of helping you lose weight, despite being so calorie rich.

Coconut oil protects your blood sugar levels

Coconut oil is a bit of a cheat in this regard. Your body burns it up immediately for fuel but, unlike a similar amount of carbohydrates, coconut oil will not spike your blood sugar and, therefore, your insulin levels.

For those battling weight gain because they have become insulin resistant, such as diabetics and anyone else caught on the inflammation/sugar addiction/fat gain roller coaster, coconut oil can nourish you without throwing your system out of whack, and without sending your body into fat-storing mode. Adding coconut oil to a meal instantly decreases its glycemic index, meaning you'll digest more steadily and store less fat.

Coconut oil is a natural appetite suppressant

It's hard to describe how deeply satiating coconut oil is when eaten regularly. If you're the kind of person who starts to fade and get "hangry" when you haven't eaten for a few hours, you may be surprised at how calm and stable you can feel after a meal with coconut oil.

Many people find skipping the occasional meal is no big deal when they eat coconut oil. Their blood sugar is stable enough and their metabolism robust enough that it simply doesn't affect them. You'll eat less and be hungry less often.

Coconut oil is the richest source of Lauric acid

Lauric acid, or more accurately, Monolaurin, literally kills viruses, bacteria, microorganisms, and fungi in the body. While leaving the beneficial gut flora intact, coconut oil flushes the body of parasites and infections.

What does this have to do with weight loss? Well, many people are completely unaware of the fact that what is keeping them from losing weight is completely unrelated to diet and exercise. As we've seen above, a Candida infection, for example, can throw everything off balance.

When your gut is overgrown with harmful bacteria, you don't have room for the good kind – the kind that makes sure you digest your food properly. Because the infection also damages your intestinal wall, you're absorbing horrible toxins into your bloodstream. This throws your hormones off balance, and quite a few hormones – Leptin and Ghrelin, for example – are responsible for your appetite and how well your body burns fat.

Add to this the Cortisol from stress and inflammation and naturally you're going to have a very hard time losing weight. With the Lauric acid in coconut oil, however, you start working at getting your body into its best working condition. You train your metabolism to burn fat instead of store it and to heal your gut so that it processes food properly.

Bloating, indigestion, heartburn, diarrhea, and constipation can all be reversed, and some of the strain on your organs in general can be reduced. Coconut oil kicks your metabolism into shape and benefits your thyroid gland and your immune system. Your body's separate systems begin to work in beautiful harmony. All of this adds up to one important thing: fat loss.

A note on polyunsaturated fatty acids

Coconut oil added on top of a terrible diet will probably not be able to work any miracles. When polyunsaturated fatty acids (PUFA) are replaced with coconut oil, the magic happens, but you need to remove harmful oils from your diet first.

PUFA in the body encourages blood clots by increasing platelet stickiness. Because these are oils rich in long chain fatty acids, they place stress on the body to digest them and are more likely stored as fat. What's more, the Omega 6 in most of these oils is not heat stable and therefore more likely to oxidize and break down when exposed to heat. The result is extra oxidation for your cells and a nasty dose of trans fatty acids.

It's crazy, but "heart friendly" oils like canola have been pushed as a smart alternative to butter, with some companies even making a canola style hydrogenated margarine. If you value your life, stay far away from these kinds of oils. Not only do they place huge oxidant loads on your body, encourage fat gain and stress your digestion, they're poor quality, too.

Here's why: Oils like safflower, sunflower, corn, canola, and soy can come from crops that are heavily treated with insecticides before being processed half to death. Fragmented, heated, deodorized, polymerized, and even colored, these oils end up on the supermarket shelf very nearly resembling poison. Eat these oils and you'll load up on potential carcinogens, solvent residue, and enough Omega 6 to throw off your 3:6 ratios.

So what oils are best?

Coconut oil is full of Omega 3s, vitamins, minerals, and the secret ingredient Lauric acid.

It's heat stable and easy on the body and can be used as energy rather than stored as fat. You could eat the bulk of your calories from coconut oil and only be leaner for it. In fact, as the old anecdote goes, farmers in the 1940s found that cheap coconut oil given to cattle didn't fatten them, but made them lean and muscular instead.

Choose fats and oils from natural, whole food sources – avocado, eggs, salmon, etc. – and stick to coconut oil, grass-fed butter, and extra virgin olive oil, used raw on salads only. And be careful with olive oil: If it mentions it is a "blend" of refined oils, that it's "light" or contains the word "pomace" anywhere, it means it's been "cut" with low quality oils or is made from the later pressings. Skip it and go for the best quality, 100% virgin olive oil instead.

What is Apple Cider Vinegar?

Let's now turn our attention to another superfood: apple cider vinegar (ACV). Apple cider vinegar is made, obviously, from apples. The apples are first crushed to extract the juice, and then bacteria and yeast can be added to ferment the sugars in the apple juice. This first fermentation is the alcoholic fermentation. It is then followed by a vinegar fermentation, where the alcohol is converted into vinegar.

The bacteria used in the second process is called acetobacter and produces acetic acid and malic acid, the things that give vinegar its characteristic taste and smell. You could then go on to pasteurize the vinegar, too. This gives the vinegar a clearer, more uniform appearance. If you leave it unpasteurized, it still contains the "mother", which is a pale cloudiness in the vinegar, sometimes resembling thin threads suspended in the clear amber liquid. You can also spot the mother as a brownish sediment on the bottom of the bottle.

Like coconut oil, apple cider vinegar is an incredibly versatile food, supplement, household cleanser, and beauty aid. Get a bottle of organic natural and unpasteurized apple cider vinegar for your pantry and you may find countless reasons to keep reaching for it.

Are all apple cider vinegars the same?

No. Like coconut oil, different vinegars differ in their nutritional content and quality.

Apple Cider Vinegar Capsules

These are often sold at health stores for the express use as weight loss aids, but the truth is there's very little you can do to find out exactly what's in these capsules. There is no regulation into what kind of vinegar you are getting and, often, some of the value is lost in the drying and powdering process. Some companies might bulk up the capsules with all sorts of weird and unusual additives. If you are certain of the quality of the capsules, however, by all means take them, especially if the taste of ACV is putting you off.

Motherless vinegar

The vinegar's mom shows herself through fine little filaments in the liquid and a kind of gross looking sediment at the bottom of the bottle. Though nothing to look at, the mother is created during the fermentation process and is full of the very enzymes and live bacteria that make ACV do its thing. Clear, golden vinegar might be prettier on the shelf, but it is simply less nutritious. Don't worry if some bottles have more mother than others – as long as you can see some of these little floating particles, the vinegar is good.

Raw, unfiltered, unheated, unprocessed, unpasteurized

This kind of vinegar is made through the fermentation processes described above, but nothing else. No colorants, flavorings, or preservatives are added. This means the final product will be a little rough looking: Individual jars from the same company may vary in color and taste, and the mother can be varied, too. But it's the best kind for its sheer nutritional value, so try to look (and smell) past its shortcomings.

Organic vs. Nonorganic

Ordinarily, the benefit of having produce grown organically is not big enough to warrant going out of your way to find it. However, there are some fruits and vegetables that, because of the way they're grown, are exposed to more pesticides. Apples are one such fruit.

Throughout their growing cycle apples are some of the most heavily sprayed and treated crops, and their thin skin means the entire fruit can become contaminated. Don't just look for "natural" or other such labels – check that the vinegar is certified organic by a credible regulating body in your area.

Plastic vs. Glass

Glass is always best but, if your vinegar is in plastic bottles, look for BPA free plastic so that it doesn't leach harmful chemicals. Darker bottles may not be as pretty, but they protect the vinegar from the sun.

Generally, if your ACV looks beautiful and sparkling yellow, has no sediment, is in a plastic bottle, and you can't glean any information from the label, it's probably of the lowest quality. ACV sold in supermarkets is usually cheap vinegar intended for salad dressings and not as a health food supplement. Buying online may be your best bet if the stores in your area don't stock good ACV.

Can I use filtered ACV for cleaning, etc.?

Absolutely. Save the better quality vinegar for drinking, and keep lower quality brands for household cleaning and using as a skin toner. However, if you use organic vinegar with a mother for your skin, the extra enzymes contained will definitely have a greater impact than would filtered vinegar.

Highly rated apple cider vinegars

Here are several excellent quality ACVs:

1. Bragg Apple Cider Vinegar

2. Omega Nutrition Certified Organic Apple Cider Vinegar – This vinegar is on the cheaper

end and comes in a black plastic container. It's advisable to decant it into a glass jar instead.

3. Vitacost Organic Apple Cider Vinegar with Mother

There are dozens of brands out there, however, and if you are satisfied that the vinegar has its mother, is unprocessed, and also not suspiciously cheap, go ahead and purchase it.

How do I store apple cider vinegar?

Because of the acidity of the vinegar, it will likely not go bad or harbor any bacteria. However, there is an expiration date on ACV that you'll need to pay attention to. Drinking bad vinegar can actually make you sick.

Refrigeration isn't necessary but keep the bottle in a dark, cool cupboard where there is enough air flow and no dampness. This will keep the vinegar's flavor strong and the health benefits intact. The vinegar will typically expire in 4 or 5 years, but will spoil if left open - bugs, dust, critters, bacteria, and fungi could invade and make the vinegar unusable.

My apple cider vinegar changed color!

Color changes are normal. After you open it, you may notice it turns cloudier, or that it changes in different weather. As long as it hasn't been stored uncovered or isn't past the expiration date, it should be perfectly fine.

Can I make my own apple cider vinegar?

Yes! If you can't get hold of good quality vinegar or simply want to try your hand at making your own, the process is easy although it does take some time.

First, take 10 organically grown apples and cut into quarters. Don't peel. Leave them to sit for a while until they turn brown, and then transfer to a glass container and cover with water. Naturally, they'll float a little. Leave in a warm, dark place for two to six months to ferment. Cover lightly with cheesecloth to keep out dust and dirt but still let the apples breath.

A scum will form on the top of the water as it ferments. There's no need to remove it. Stir weekly to keep things even. Some ferment for only half this time, but they'll get a more diluted vinegar. After the time is up, strain through the same cheesecloth and let the mixture sit for another two to six months. You'll have organic, homemade, unfiltered apple cider vinegar with the mother, ready to consume.

Here's a tip: Once the vinegar is made, store in pretty glass bottles with added garlic cloves, sprigs of rosemary or a single dried chili pepper. This flavors the vinegar and can make a lovely gift for friends and family.

What Apple Cider Vinegar Can Do For You

Here are some great, easy ways to start using apple cider vinegar in your everyday life:

• ACV makes an excellent hair rinse. Combine a teaspoon or two in a jug of water and rinse through the hair after shampooing. The vinegar softens and smoothes, detangles, and leaves a serious shine afterwards, particularly with dark hair. Experiment with a rinse of brewed nettle tea, a few drops of rosemary oil and ACV – all of this turns up the shine and can leave hair very glossy. And don't worry about the smell at all – once your hair is dry and styled the smell will evaporate. Try this treatment once a week or as often as desired. It will also soften the scalp and reduce dandruff.

• Apple cider vinegar makes a good skin toner. It balances the pH level of the skin, so is a great tonic to wipe over the face with a cotton ball after cleansing and before moisturizing. It's great for balancing combination skins – softening dry areas and drying out oily patches. Don't use it neat though: Create a mix of ⅓ water and ⅔ ACV and apply only a thin film. Pure witch hazel and a few drops of lavender oil in this mixture will tighten, tone, and soothe redness as well.

• ACV can fade age spots and acne scars, as well as dry out active acne pustules, whiteheads, and blackheads. Dab the tiniest drop onto affected areas before bed every night.

• Dip your finger into pure ACV and rub over the teeth to remove coffee and tea stains and to help fade yellowness. Remember to rinse with water afterwards.

• Soak in a bath with a cup of apple cider vinegar added to soothe bad sunburn. You could also throw in a blob of coconut oil, too, or spread a thin, healing layer on the burnt area afterwards.

• Soaking calloused, tired feet in a diluted apple cider vinegar solution will soften dry skin and make it easier to slough off dead skin cells.

• Ticks and fleas really hate ACV, so use this to your advantage by making a weak ACV rinse to dip your dog in after shampooing. Otherwise, you could massage the vinegar directly into the skin or spritz the fur with a homemade ACV solution. One application is not enough though. You will need to keep it up to make sure that all the eggs, larvae, and adults are thoroughly eliminated from the coat.

• ACV is a brilliant household cleaner that is natural and free from allergy causing chemicals. Mix ½ cup of ACV to 1 cup water and use this with a cloth or sponge to clean the entire kitchen or bathroom. It's great for breaking down mold in showers, degreasing appliances, cleaning mirrors, surfaces, or windows, and wiping down refrigerators or microwaves.

• Pour apple cider vinegar into the toilet and let it sit for a while to kill germs, remove stains, and freshen your bathroom. When you flush, it'll smell faintly of apples!

• A tiny jar of ACV placed in the back of your fridge will absorb smells and keep things fresh. Likewise, the odor-eliminating power of ACV makes it great for rinsing carpets and rugs, washing down ovens and cooktops, or cleaning things like blenders and Tupperware, which can often collect smells over time.

• Drench the inside of a small adhesive bandage with ACV and apply to a wart to help remove it.

• Let dentures soak overnight in a solution of water and ACV – it will kill bacteria, remove odors, and help to whiten.

• Apply ACV-soaked bandages to bruises to reduce swelling and promote healing.

Darrin Wiggins

The Fat Burning Power of Apple Cider Vinegar

Several studies have found that apple cider vinegar has fat burning properties, but one of the most popular was conducted in Japan. Obese participants were sorted into three groups. One group was given a 500-ml drink containing 30 milliliters of AVC, the other group 15 milliliters, and the last group had the drink without any ACV in it. Each group had to drink this mix daily for twelve weeks along with controlled diets and identical levels of exercise.

After the experiment was over, the groups that drank the apple cider vinegar drinks had lower body mass indexes, less visceral fat, lower waist circumference measurements, improved serum triglyceride levels, and lower total body weight than the group that drank no ACV. Over the study period, the participants in the first two groups lost around 1 or 2 kilograms (2-4 pounds), which is modest, but potentially significant over longer periods of time.

Remember, these groups ate no differently than the control group and did the same amount of exercise, so the weight loss was due to the ACV alone. While the weight loss was gradual in this study, it may be preferable to losing a lot of weight over a short period of time and merely gaining it back again. Losing weight slowly normally means you keep it off in the future.

How exactly does apple cider vinegar help you lose weight?

Apple cider vinegar contains pectin

Pectin is a natural source of dietary fiber commonly found in apples. Apple cider vinegar contains high amounts of pectin but, unlike eating fresh apples, it doesn't come with a hefty dose of fruit sugars included. This means you can get the healthy boost of fiber from pectin without added calories or the insulin spike. Pectin helps keep you feeling full and satisfied, and over time contributes to a regulated appetite and eating less at each meal.

Apple cider vinegar improves digestion

The Malic and Acetic acid in apple cider vinegar are excellent at breaking down protein in the body and aiding in efficient digestion and absorption of amino acids. Every process that relies on the synthesis of these amino acids into hormones and enzymes is improved by apple cider vinegar.

For example, growth hormone relies on the proper breakdown and resynthesis of protein in the body. With growth hormone's help, the body processes fat more efficiently. Your digestion is streamlined and the metabolism given healthy stimulation to burn food more efficiently. Problems can arise when food sits for too long in the digestive tract, and fats have more opportunity to be absorbed and stored. However with apple cider vinegar, the digestion process is quickened, letting your body absorb what it needs and expelling what it doesn't.

Apple cider vinegar aids iron absorption and contains plenty of potassium

The acids in ACV help release the iron from your food, and iron is especially valuable when it comes to building hemoglobin and myoglobin in your blood. When all of these processes are working at their peak, the metabolism and use of oxygen is enhanced, and weight loss is indirectly supported.

Potassium, on the other hand, is a vital nutrient needed by the body to balance out sodium levels. A diet high in salt means you'll carry more bloating and water weight, as well as crave more fatty and sweet foods. ACV balances the salt in your body and reduces your appetite for junk food. In fact by simply adding ACV to your recipes, you'll find you need less salt.

Apple cider vinegar lowers blood sugar levels

ACV interferes with your body's ability to digest starch. This means you're less likely to get that spike in blood sugar and the corresponding insulin spike. When blood sugar levels are stable and insulin production more gradual, you're less likely to pack away excess energy as fat, less likely to disrupt hunger and fat-storing hormones, and less likely to experience cravings, inflammation, hunger, and sugar "crashes" as your blood sugar levels adjust. All in all, more stable blood sugar levels = less stored fat.

Using apple cider vinegar

The good thing about apple cider vinegar is that you only need a little to notice the effects. It's easy to sneak into your everyday diet and only a few teaspoons will do the trick. Here are some ways to get apple cider vinegar into your daily life.

For weight loss

Apple cider vinegar is best avoided on an empty stomach. Instead, pair it with food, preferably before a meal. ACV eaten before breakfast, lunch, and dinner will lower the effective GI of the foods you eat, add to feelings of satiety, and keep your blood sugar nice and regular.

Aim for around one to two teaspoons before meals. You can drink it just like that or, better yet, add it to a glass of water. Others find it easier to just incorporate the vinegar directly into their meals. Try starting dinner with a small side salad dressed with olive oil and ACV.

Sprinkle over roast potatoes and vegetables or add it to sauces. Vinegar actually enhances the taste of food and brings out the salty, savory taste. Chefs are taught to add acids like lemon juice and vinegar to salty foods as they sharpen each other's flavor. You'll use less salt as a result.

Ewww! What do I do if I hate the taste?

Good quality apple cider vinegar tastes just like you'd expect – like regular vinegar with a fresh hint of apple juice. Many people love sour and vinegary tastes, but others want to retch at the idea of eating it at all.

First of all, different vinegars will have different acidity levels, and if you find one with 5 or 6% acidity, you may find the taste more palatable. If experimenting with different brands doesn't work, your next option is to dilute the vinegar quite a bit. Many recommend drinking the vinegar down with plenty of water to mask the taste, but whether you want all your water to taste mildly sour is neither here nor there.

Hiding ACV in regular dressings is a good idea, as the oil balances out the sourness. Try taking smaller amounts more often, or you could even try pickling vegetables in the vinegar. If need be, just hold your nose and swallow! Of course, a really bad taste could indicate that your vinegar is a poor quality brand or just plain off.

Precautions and realistic expectations

ACV works as a weight loss tonic, but there's nothing instant about it. Losing weight with ACV is more about slowly and steadily winning the race. Keep up your daily intake and you will notice the weight shifting, although it will happen slowly, that is, over the course of months rather than weeks.

Take heart though – the weight you lose typically stays off for good. Your body's metabolism has time to adapt and adjust slowly, so you're not just on a roller-coaster of water weight loss and gain. Plus, adding ACV to your daily life gives you a host of other health benefits, too. You'll lose weight, but in the long term you'll have a more robust, healthy metabolism and digestive system.

If you are considering ingesting it on a regular basis keep in mind that it is very acidic. It is a good idea to dilute it with water or juice as long term use can potentially damage the tissue in your mouth and throat. This may only be in extreme cases, but you should be aware of it.

Be careful that the ACV doesn't have too much time to wear away at the tooth enamel, either. If you rub some on your teeth, follow with plain water to rinse, and if you have a lot of ACV at one time, try to rinse your mouth afterwards or even brush your teeth. Coconut oil taken regularly will help counter the acid in ACV.

If you tolerate acids well, this may not be much of a problem, but on the whole it's better to consume the bulk of your ACV with other foods, or diluted with water. ACV is indeed a powerful food supplement, but it still is a food. It's not necessary to force yourself to swallow it down neat if you can find functional ways to incorporate it into recipes without even noticing.

This is especially necessary if you suffer from GERD (extreme reflux and heartburn), ulcers, or digestive disorders. Start small and notice how your body reacts. The fact is many people claim to actually reverse poor digestion and heartburn by slowly introducing ACV into their diets. Try it and see.

Darrin Wiggins

Mother Nature's Weight Loss Duo

Now that we've seen the weight loss and wellness powers of both coconut oil and apple cider vinegar, we can see how well they work together and how they are natural allies in regaining your health, burning fat, and getting your entire system in peak working condition:

• Both coconut oil and apple cider vinegar work together to normalize blood sugar levels. Coconut oil is an easily digested fat that requires no insulin production, and ACV slows the digestion of the foods with which it's paired, lowering the glycemic index and providing appetite suppressing fiber.

• Both will work synergistically to get your appetite under control, to reduce cravings and improve the digestion. While coconut oil heals the inner lining of the intestine, ACV speeds and enhances the passage of food. This means that poor digestion, bloating, gas, discomfort, reflux, and nausea are reduced by the ACV and healed and soothed by the coconut oil.

• Both of these healthy miracle foods will destroy bacteria and parasites in the digestive system, balance pH levels and help restore the inner gut flora. You'll kill excessive Candida and helicobacter populations, soothe ulcers and leaky gut as well as prevent future onset, and regulate blood sugar, insulin production, and hunger.

• When used together, both coconut oil and apple cider vinegar can prove to be a potent combination for taking charge of your digestion, your weight, your immune system and, ultimately, your well-being.

So many people have come to realize that radiant health is something they, too, deserve, without it being a question of taking synthetic, side-effect-causing medications that only mask the symptoms. After years of battling misdiagnosis, of being thrown out of balance by antibiotics, of feeling as though they are always fighting against the body and never working with it, some people are nothing less than astonished that true health was so close at hand, and never required anything more than natural, wholesome food supplements.

Both coconut oil and ACV can be easily incorporated into any diet, and can replace foods that are not actually working for your body. Health and wellness are about making choices that truly serve you. The process of becoming unhealthy is a long one and the road back to good health takes time too.

It won't make much sense to add coconut oil and apple cider vinegar to your diet while still eating other foods that undermine your health. Here are some harmful foods that can be gradually replaced with coconut oil and ACV.

Margarine

More or less edible plastic, don't ever buy margarine, no matter how many heart logos you see on the tub. Use olive oil, real butter, or coconut oil instead.

Soda and blended fruit juices

Sugar shouldn't be thought of as a food group, but rather almost like a condiment – something nice to add here and there, but never the staple of an entire meal. There is nothing good about soda and no way to drink it healthfully. Artificial sweeteners have their own host of health problems, too. If you're craving something soda-like, try this recipe for a refreshing and healthy homemade drink: mix a teaspoon of baking soda, a wedge of lemon and a teaspoon of apple cider vinegar. This is a cleansing, refreshing, and alkalizing drink that will also help with indigestion and heartburn.

When it comes to fruit juice, most of the time you're consuming pure sugar with very little fiber and only traces of the original vitamins and minerals left after processing. Many people simply imagine that fruit juice is made by crushing the relevant fruit and bottling the juice, but in fact many juices, for example orange juice, are pulverized, loaded with preservatives, and often stored in enormous vats for years.

To reconstitute it, orange color and orange flavoring is added, and dry pulp from previously juiced oranges is added too, to give it that "freshly squeezed" look. If you crave something sweet, eat an actual fruit so you benefit from the fiber, but resist marketing that pushes fruit juices as healthy.

Creamy sauces, mayonnaise, thousand island or ranch style dressings, etc.

You'd be horrified to spend a day at the salad dressing factory. A bland, tasteless base of thickeners and emulsifiers is blended with poor quality vegetable oil and laced with salt, MSG, and nasty flavorings. "Diet" or reduced calorie varieties are the worst as they contain terrible oils – canola and sunflower seed are the usual culprits – and extra sugar.

As a rule, don't trust store-bought or restaurant dressings, no matter how innocuous they seem. Stick to things like lemon juice, good quality balsamic vinegar, apple cider or rice wine vinegar, extra virgin olive oil, and real mayonnaise made with olive oil and egg yolks.

Lastly, opt for whole milk and not skim or 2%, choose whole cuts of meat rather than processed meats like sausages or chicken nuggets, eat whole eggs and not just the whites, drink plenty of water, reduce the amount of grains and legumes and increase the calories you get from vegetable carbohydrates, and make sure that at every meal you are getting quality fats and proteins.

Do all of this and you'll enhance the fat burning and metabolism boosting effects of the coconut oil and ACV.

The apple cider vinegar and coconut oil weight loss cleanse

If you're confident you have eliminated most unwholesome foods from your refrigerator and pantry, you can kick off some new healthy habits by engaging in a deliberate cleanse/fast. If your body has experienced a whole lifetime of bad habits and toxic foods, it may be a bit difficult to start out on a healthier path – but it's definitely worth it.

A simple 3-day cleanse

For those who are not used to coconut oil or ACV, start small. This is important: You will gain no benefit by jumping in immediately to do a fast/cleanse that your body is not prepare for. Again, it is not a question of willpower, but of doing what is right for your body wherever it is on its journey.

This first cleanse is a great way to start. You will not be reducing calories or eating differently. Maintain your normal (good) diet, but add 3 tablespoons of coconut oil as well as a tablespoon of ACV a day. You can choose how you'd like to do this, but around mealtimes is best.

This will prepare your body and get it used to the effects of both ACV and coconut oil so that you don't shock your system when you attempt a longer fast/cleanse.

The 3-day fat fast

To call this a fast is a bit misleading, as you will not be reducing calories – only taking your calories in fat form. First calculate your daily caloric requirements, more or less. There are approximately 117 calories in a tablespoon of coconut oil, and the average woman needs around 1200 to 1700 calories a day.

This means that, throughout the day, you will be consuming anywhere between 10 and 14 tablespoons of coconut oil. That's a lot! For this reason, don't attempt a 3-day fat fast if you are not comfortable with eating at least 3 tablespoons a day with no problem.

If you just jump right in and eat 14 tablespoons, you'll end up nauseous or vomiting, not to mention running to the bathroom about 50 times a day. But if your body is used to it, a coconut oil fat fast will starve off Candida overgrowth, kickstart serious fat burning, and give your digestive system a break.

While you complete the fast, take plenty of water with at least two teaspoons of diluted apple cider vinegar. If you find yourself needing a bit of extra nourishment, an egg, a small handful of macadamia nuts or a small serving of pure protein can be taken to help keep you on track. If the sheer volume of coconut oil seems overwhelming, listen to your body and only take as much as you can manage. It's only three days, so you will not do any damage to your muscles and will not starve.

The 7-day fat fast

If you have completed a 3-day fat fast comfortably, you can start to extend the time you spend on coconut oil and ACV alone. Always listen to your body. Flu-like symptoms, crabbiness, fatigue, headaches, and listlessness are all normal detox symptoms, so try to stick it out. If you faint or have serious issues maintaining energy, there's nothing wrong with stopping and reverting to a gentler cleanse for the remaining days.

Your own personal detox

There are no hard and fast rules, though, and when it comes to incorporating healthy habits into your life, it's all about what works for you. You may find a seven-day cleanse is easier to complete if you have some low-calorie crunchy vegetables or soup to eat throughout the day. Or perhaps you don't need a cleanse so much as to just eliminate bad foods from your diet and add more healing and beneficial ones.

Your body is a sophisticated and complex machine that will tell you whether something is helping or harming. Listen closely and adjust as you see fit, so that you maintain your lifestyle and respect your own limits.

Sample Meal Plan

Having considered a few ways to make adjustments to our diet, here is a possible diet plan you can follow to incorporate both apple cider vinegar and coconut oil into your life. It's nutritionally balanced and lets you easily include both of these superfoods. This is a good long term approach and will help you reach your weight loss and health goals gradually but permanently. Adjust it as you feel necessary.

On Waking

Start your morning with a coconut oil pull for 3 days a week, otherwise take a spoonful of the oil in a cup of herbal tea of your choice.

Breakfast

A few hours after waking, eat a breakfast of steel cut oats, a handful of blueberries, and a boiled egg for protein. Have with a good cup of coffee blended with coconut oil and a little full fat cream. This breakfast will give you plenty of energy to last way past lunch time. Fiber, vitamins and minerals, and a good shot of both healthy fat and protein will keep your blood sugar levels constant. If it's your preference, you may also fast for breakfast.

Snack

It's really not necessary to have snacks throughout the day, and the idea that our metabolism will be boosted this way is a bit of an old wives' tale. If you get peckish, have a drink of 1 teaspoon baking soda, a teaspoon of apple cider vinegar, and a wedge of lemon in a glass of water to refresh you, or else have a small handful of nuts or a protein shake blended with a little coconut oil. Avoid fruit.

Lunch

Make an enormous salad with any and all veggies you can find. Load up your plate with lettuce, tomato, cucumber, onion, peppers, pickles, boiled eggs, chicken or ham, tuna or salmon pieces, nuts, seeds, berries, tofu, and whatever else looks good. Next, whisk together some extra virgin olive oil with an equal amount of ACV, add dried herbs, salt and pepper to season, and drizzle over the salad. Finish off with a spoon of coconut oil to keep you sated and happy until dinner. Have tea, coffee, diluted fruit or vegetable juice, or coconut water to keep hydrated throughout the day.

Dinner

You could start your dinner with an appetizer of side salad with the same dressing as with lunch, or have a glass of water with the apple cider vinegar just before you eat to curb appetite and ease digestion. For dinner, have a serving of protein at least the size and thickness of your palm – try salmon or tuna medallions, grass-fed steak, whole fish (like mackerel or pilchards), two pieces of chicken, or a slice of gammon ham. Pile up the rest of the plate with steamed vegetables, roasted sweet potato or pumpkin. You can cook with the coconut oil or, if the taste would be distracting, save it for dessert.

Dessert

Have some stewed fruit with cinnamon and a teaspoon of raw honey drizzled over it for a special treat, or whip some cream with a half teaspoon of fine sugar and serve over fresh strawberries. See the recipe below for coconut oil "fat bombs", a delicious and nutritious snack or dessert.

Recipes

Basic apple cider vinaigrette

Whisk ½ cup ACV with ½ cup olive oil until emulsified. Add one teaspoon each of chopped fresh herbs: mint, parsley, and cilantro. Add salt and pepper to taste.

Creamy dressing

Mix ½ cup of plain Greek or Bulgarian yogurt with 2 teaspoons ACV, 1 tablespoon of olive oil, and 1 tablespoon of finely diced red onion. Add 1 mashed hardboiled egg. This is a great substitute for creamy ranch-style dressings and tastes just as good – or better.

Coconut oil "fat bombs"

Mix a cup of desiccated coconut with a teaspoon of raw or manuka honey, 2 teaspoons cocoa powder, 2 tablespoons of melted or soft coconut oil, a dash of cinnamon, ½ teaspoons of vanilla essence, and the tiniest pinch of salt. Adjust the quantities to make a sort of stiff "dough", roll into truffle sized balls, and then coat in more desiccated coconut and set in the refrigerator for a few hours.

These are endlessly versatile and can be made with whatever you have on hand – finely chopped fresh dates or cranberries; flax seeds; chopped nuts; fresh blueberries; macadamia, peanut, or almond butter; tahini or almond flour; or even add a little grated dark chocolate. Just go wild and when you get the right consistency and roll away.

These are great for little snacks during the day, with a cup of coffee, or as a dessert. You may even find you come up with a combo that's so good you eat them all up immediately!

Thai style coconut soup

The Thai know how to use coconut better than anyone, so a Thai cookbook is a great place to start for inspiration to use coconut in all its wonderful forms. Here's an easy and nutritious soup that can be adapted depending on what you have.

Heat a diced onion and a thumb-sized knob of finely diced fresh ginger in a big pot and then add 4 sliced chicken breasts or else some thin slices of beef. Add some sliced shiitake mushrooms, grated carrots and a handful of bean sprouts. Stir fry for a few moments, adding a dash of soy sauce and fish sauce, about a teaspoon each.

When the vegetables are a little softened, add a can of coconut milk, the same volume of chicken or vegetable stock, a tablespoon of turmeric, a tablespoon of coconut oil, and a tablespoon of lime juice. Turn down the heat and allow to simmer for 15 to 20 minutes. Serve with rice noodles, basmati rice, or alone as a soup and garnish with a squeeze of lemon and some fresh chopped cilantro. In one bowl, you'll get a healthy serving of veggies, fat, and protein. And it tastes amazing

Conclusion

There is something infinitely pleasing in paring down your eating, health, and beauty routines to only the most effective natural ingredients. Sadly, our modern consumer culture encourages us to go out and buy a million different chemical-laden and environmentally damaging products that, frankly, only work some of the time. Rather than being for our best health and well-being, these products are heavily marketed to appeal to our weakness and ego, and whether they respect our bodies' natural balance is not really anyone's concern.

But with natural food supplements, you can begin to gently and effectively take charge of your health and well-being, lose weight and reverse health conditions that conventional medicine cannot. With the amazing healing, balancing, and vitalizing effects of both coconut oil and apple cider vinegar, you can take charge of your body and give it the opportunity to fulfil its inborn purpose: to be strong, dynamic, and brimming with vitality.

Both coconut oil and apple cider vinegar have been proven to work synergistically with one another, helping your body burn fat, digest with ease, and heal from the inside out. And you'll find dozens of other applications the longer you keep these two superstars in your kitchen cupboard.

What can coconut oil and apple cider vinegar do for you on your weight loss and wellness journey?

Darrin Wiggins

One last thing….

If you feel this book has added value to your life I would appreciate you taking the time to leave an honest review on Amazon for me.

I cherish people's feedback as it allows me to continue growing as a person. Reviews also help people make informed decisions about the action they are about to take and taking action is what I am all about.

Thank you for taking the time to read my book. I hope it has improved the quality of your life.

About The Author

Darrin Wiggins is a best-selling weight loss and self-help author who has a passion for helping people change their lives. He spent over a decade helping people improve the quality of their life through goal coaching them to become more than they believed possible. He wanted to find a way to reach more people so he decided to share his knowledge by becoming a full-time writer.

The passion for personal development books comes from the results he saw people getting with the goal setting work they were doing. Ordinary people were creating the lives of their dreams by focusing on their goals. By following the advice of the greats like Tony Robbins and Brian Tracy, Darrin now enjoys the life many people only dream of.

His interest in weight loss turned into a passion after he lost 45 pounds in 12 weeks healthily and naturally by customizing a diet for himself. His personal weight loss success is the driving force

Darrin Wiggins

behind the weight loss books he writes today. There is a diet out there that will give you the results you are looking for, but it takes trial and error.

By combining self-help, goal setting and weight loss, people can tackle the internal issues that typically cause weight gain in the first place. Once a person discovers why they eat the way they eat, they can start the healing process and then focus on diet. Trying to lose weight when you are not emotionally healthy does not usually end with success. Once they combine emotional health and diet with goal setting there really is nothing they cannot accomplish both with their body and their life.

He hopes his books truly inspire people to live healthy, think wealthy and discover their own definition of happiness. The life of your dreams is inside you and you deserve to live it.

http://www.amazon.com/Darrin-Wiggins/e/B00BPEPGYU/

Preview of Fruit Infused Water: 70 Vitamin Water Recipes To Finally Cure Tasteless H2O

Chapter 1 Delicious Weight Loss Medleys

Vitamin C is a great metabolism booster and most of these recipes will give you a healthy dose of it. You will also be protecting your health with the antioxidants found in these drinks.

Garden Delight

Ingredients:

½ cucumber, medium (sliced)

¼ cantaloupe (cubed)

¼ honeydew melon (cubed)

Directions:

Remove the rind from the cantaloupe and honeydew and cut into cubes. Add the fruit to your one quart jar.

Take your muddler or wooden spoon and press the fruit so it starts to release its juices. You want to "break them open" without turning them into a paste.

Now fill the jar three quarters full of ice and top off with water if you are letting it sit overnight. If you want to consume within the next three to five hours fill the jar half full of ice and then top off with cold water.

Put the lid on your jar and place in the fridge for desired length of time.

Strain before serving.

Blackberry Lime Water

Ingredients:

2 slices orange

3 slices lime

10 blackberries

Directions:

Add the fruit to your one quart jar.

Take your muddler or wooden spoon and press the fruit so it starts to release its juices. You want to "break them open" without turning them into a paste.

Now fill the jar three quarters full of ice and top off with water if you are letting it sit overnight. If you want to consume within the next three to five hours fill the jar half full of ice and then top off with cold water.

Put the lid on your jar and place in the fridge for desired length of time.

Strain before serving.

Lemony Blueberry

10 blueberries

1 lemon slice

2 orange slices

Directions:

Add the fruit to your one quart jar.

Take your muddler or wooden spoon and press the fruit so it starts to release its juices. You want to "break them open" without turning them into a paste.

Now fill the jar three quarters full of ice and top off with water if you are letting it sit overnight. If you want to consume within the next three to five hours fill the jar half full of ice and then top off with cold water.

Put the lid on your jar and place in the fridge for desired length of time.

Strain before serving.

Berry Tasty Water

Ingredients:

½ c. blueberries

½ c. raspberries

½ c. cherries

Directions:

Remove the pits from the cherries. Add the fruit to your one quart jar.

Take your muddler or wooden spoon and press the fruit so it starts to release its juices. You want to "break them open" without turning them into a paste.

Now fill the jar three quarters full of ice and top off with water if you are letting it sit overnight. If you want to consume within the next three to five hours fill the jar half full of ice and then top off with cold water.

Put the lid on your jar and place in the fridge for desired length of time.

Strain before serving.

Tart Delight

Ingredients:

½ c. cherries

4 cubes watermelon

5 strawberries (sliced)

Directions:

Remove the tops of the strawberries, rind from the watermelon and pits from cherries. Add the fruit to your one quart jar.

Take your muddler or wooden spoon and press the fruit so it starts to release its juices. You want to "break them open" without turning them into a paste.

Now fill the jar three quarters full of ice and top off with water if you are letting it sit overnight. If you want to consume within the next three to five hours fill the jar half full of ice and then top off with cold water.

Put the lid on your jar and place in the fridge for desired length of time.

Strain before serving.

Tropical Paradise

Ingredients:

1 mango (cored and peeled)

1 orange (peeled and sliced)

½ c. pineapple (chunks)

Directions:

Add the fruit to your one quart jar.

Take your muddler or wooden spoon and press the fruit so it starts to release its juices. You want to "break them open" without turning them into a paste.

Now fill the jar three quarters full of ice and top off with water if you are letting it sit overnight. If you want to consume within the next three to five hours fill the jar half full of ice and then top off with cold water.

Put the lid on your jar and place in the fridge for desired length of time.

Strain before serving.

END OF PREVIEW

To view the entire book, click the link below.

Darrin Wiggins

http://amzn.to/1m99EgH

Copyright/Disclaimer

Copyright 2014 by Darrin Wiggins - All rights reserved.

This document is geared towards providing exact and reliable information in regards to the topic and issue covered. The publication is sold with the idea that the publisher is not required to render accounting, officially permitted, or otherwise, qualified services. If advice is necessary, legal or professional, a practiced individual in the profession should be ordered.

- From a Declaration of Principles which was accepted and approved equally by a Committee of the American Bar Association and a Committee of Publishers and Associations.

The information provided herein is stated to be truthful and consistent, in that any liability, in terms of inattention or otherwise, by any usage or abuse of any policies, processes, or directions contained within is the solitary and utter responsibility of the recipient reader. Under no circumstances will any legal responsibility or blame be held against the publisher for any reparation, damages, or monetary loss due to the information herein, either directly or indirectly.

The information provided in this book is for educational and entertainment purposes only. The author is not a physician and this is not to be taken as medical advice or a recommendation to stop taking medications. The information provided in this book is based on the author's experiences and interpretations of the past and current research available. You should consult your physician to insure the daily habits and principles in this book are appropriate for your individual circumstances. If you have any health issues or pre-existing conditions, please consult your doctor before implementing any of the information you have learned in this book. Results will vary from individual to individual. This book is for informational purposes only and the author does not accept any responsibilities for any liabilities or damages, real or perceived, resulting from the use of this information.

The information herein is offered for informational purposes solely, and is universal as so. The presentation of the information is without contract or any type of guarantee assurance.

The trademarks that are used are without any consent, and the publication of the trademark is without permission or backing by the trademark owner. All trademarks and brands within this book are for clarifying purposes only and are owned by the owners themselves, not affiliated with this document.

Darrin Wiggins

References

Here are some studies and reviews done on the efficacy of coconut oil and apple cider vinegar and on weight loss and general well-being:

• de Lourdes Arruzazabala, M.; Molina, V.; Más, R.; Carbajal, D.; Marrero, D.; González, V.; Rodríguez, E. (2007). "Effects of coconut oil on testosterone-induced prostatic hyperplasia in Sprague-Dawley rats." Journal of Pharmacy and Pharmacology 59 (7): 995–999. doi:10.1211/jpp.59.7.0012. PMID 17637195. edit.

• Nevin, K.G.; Rajamohan, T. "Beneficial effects of virgin coconut oil on lipid parameters and in vitro LDL oxidation." Clinical Biochemistry. 37(9):830-5, 2004 Sep. [Comparative Study. Journal Article] UI: 15329324.

• Khonkarn, R.; Okonogi, S.; Ampasavate, C.; Anuchapreeda, S. "Investigation of fruit peel extracts as sources for compounds with antioxidant and antiproliferative activities against human cell lines." Food & Chemical Toxicology. 48(8-9):2122-9, 2010 Aug-Sep.

[Journal Article. Research Support, Non-U.S. Gov't] UI: 20510336.

• Radenahmad, N.; Saleh, F.; Sawangjaroen, K.; Rundorn, W.; Withyachumnarnkul, B.; Connor, J.R. "Young coconut juice significantly reduces histopathological changes in the brain that are induced by hormonal imbalance: a possible implication to postmenopausal women." Histology & Histopathology. 24(6):667-74, 2009 Jun. [Journal Article. Research Support, Non-U.S. Gov't] UI: 19337965.

• Eiseman, B.; Lozano, R.E.; Hager, T. "Clinical Experience in Intravenous Administration of Coconut Water." In A.M.A. Archives of Surgery, 1954.

• Campbell-Falck, D.; Thomas, T.; Falck, T.M.; Tutuo, N.; Clem K. "The intravenous use of coconut water." American Journal of Emergency Medicine. 18(1):108-11, 2000 Jan. [Case Reports. Journal Article] UI: 10674546.

• Rinaldi, S.; Silva, D. O.; Bello, F.; Alviano, C. S.; Alviano, D. S.; Matheus, M. E.; Fernandes, P. D. "Characterization of the antinociceptive and anti-inflammatory activities from Cocos nucifera L. (Palmae)." Journal of Ethnopharmacology 122 (3): 541–546. doi:10.1016/j.jep.2009.01.024. PMID 19429325.

• Chambers, Ruth; Wakley, Gill. "History of over the counter medicines." Obesity and Overweight Matters in Primary Care, Radcliffe Publishing (2002), p. 101.

• Knight, Charles (1867). "Obesity." The English Cyclopaedia, 4 "Arts and Sciences," Bradbury, Evans, pp. 12–13.

• Östman, J; Britton, M, eds. (2004). "4.7.3 Alternative Medicine Methods Used to Treat Obesity." Treating and Preventing Obesity: An Evidence Based Review, Wiley-VCH, pp. 202–204.

• Kondo, Tomoo; Kishi, Mikiya; Fushimi, Takashi; Kaga, Takayuki (2009). "Acetic Acid Upregulates the Expression of Genes for Fatty Acid Oxidation Enzymes in Liver To Suppress Body Fat Accumulation." J. Agric. Food Chem. 57 (13): 5982–5986, doi:10.1021/jf900470c.

- Kondo, Tomoo, et al.; Kishi, Mikiya; Fushimi, Takashi; Ugajin, Shinobu; Kaga, Takayuki (2009). "Vinegar Intake Reduces Body Weight, Body Fat Mass, and Serum Triglyceride Levels in Obese Japanese Subjects." Bioscience, Biotechnology, and Biochemistry 73 (8): 1837–1843. doi:10.1271/bbb.90231. PMID 19661687. Retrieved 15 Mar 2013.

Made in the USA
Columbia, SC
31 March 2018